DASH Diet

Delicious DASH Diet Recipes to Lose Weight Naturally, Lower Blood Pressure and Live Healthy- Includes 7-day Meal Plan

By

Anne Wilson

TABLE OF CONTENTS

Introduction..iv

FREE Bonus Offer:..v

Chapter 1: DASH Diet to Shrink the Waistline 1

Chapter 2: DASH Food Groups and Recommended Servings...........6

Chapter 3: Breakfast DASH Recipes...12

Chapter 4: Lunch DASH Recipes...28

Chapter 5: Dinner DASH Recipes 46

Chapter 6: Snack DASH Recipes 63

Chapter 7: Sample 7-Day DASH Diet Meal Plan...........................78

Conclusion 93

INTRODUCTION

I want to thank you and congratulate you for purchasing the book DASH Diet: Delicious DASH Diet Recipes to Lose Weight Naturally, Lower Blood Pressure and Live Healthy- Includes 7-Day Meal Plan

This book contains proven steps and strategies on how to become a truly healthy person. You can lose excess weight and have a slimmer waistline without starving yourself to death. This isn't a yo-yo or a fad diet that gives instant result but will give you more problems later on.

Here's an inescapable fact: you will need to be more conscious of the things you eat. There is also some level of sacrifice required from you in order to change your dietary practices and lifestyle into something healthier.

If you do not develop a good knowledge and understanding of the proper diet, you may end up harming your body more. People who do not understand that food is the main factor that determines how much you weigh, weight loss will never be of a satisfying level.

It's time for you to become an amazingly fit and healthier individual. This book will show you the guidelines on how to lose excess weight and trim down your waist in a healthy yet effective manner. This book will also show you recipes that prove proper diet can be both healthy and delicious.

YOUR FREE GIFT:

As a way of saying thanks for your purchase, I am offering a free report that's exclusive to my book readers.

With 45 Fantastic Ways To Burn Calories you'll discover easy to follow calorie-burning secrets that will ramp up your metabolism and help you become slimmer, fitter and happier

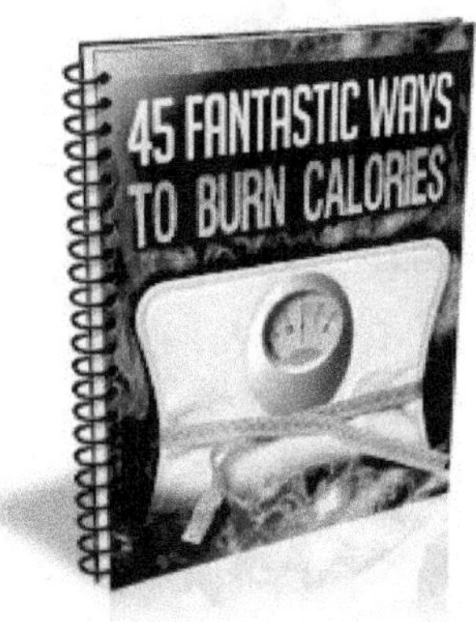

http://www.weightlossbonusguide.com/

CHAPTER 1

DASH DIET TO SHRINK THE WAISTLINE

The DASH diet safely follows 2 phases. The diet plan starts with a 14-day Phase 1 that helps regulate blood sugar levels. Properly satisfying hunger and dealing with cravings are also important goals in this phase.

The next stage, Phase 2, is making DASH diet a lifestyle. DASH diet is not a one-time only thing to meet your health and fitness goals. Yes, it is effective to achieve slimmer waistlines in a shorter amount of time. However, the best results for both your waistline and your overall health are achieved when you make DASH diet a lifestyle. That said, Phase 2 is changing the way you see and treat food and eating as a whole.

DASH for weight loss Phase 1

This is the first 2 weeks of the diet that will help you lose a lot of excess fats around your waistline. This is also the period where you will be lighter and feel lighter as well.

The most important part of this phase is to avoid starchy food that contain lots of sugar. The major effect of this dietary change is to regulate your blood sugar level. That alone will create a long list of benefits such as:

- Improved insulin control
- Effectively controls cravings
- Have more energy
- Regulate hunger better
- Feel fuller longer
- Heighten fat metabolism
- Improve heart health
- Improve circulation
- Improve cognitive abilities (ability to think, decide, etc.)
- Better mood control

And the list goes on.

At this time, you will be concentrating on eating more leafy greens and cruciferous vegetables. You will have to avoid whole grains and fruits at this time, too because of the high amounts of natural sugars.

Phase 1 would essentially be about fresh salads with low-sodium, low-fat dressings. Yogurt will be your best friend when it comes to salad dressings.

Meats and other healthy sources of proteins are allowed during Phase 1. If you get tired of green salads, you can go for bread-less sandwiches. Think: lean burger with low fat dressing, lots of vegetables like tomatoes and cabbages, no ketchup, no buns and no cheese.

This phase is also your opportunity to try eating seafood such as wild salmon and tuna. Poultry is also good.

Losing a few inches does not have to be boring salads day in and day out. You can enjoy eating still. You just have to sacrifice your pasta, breads, toasts, bagels and other starchy food. No cake, too. But hey, what's giving up a slice of cake for looking good in clothes 2 to 3 sizes smaller than what you are wearing today?

The basics of Phase 1 are:

- No starchy food
- Nothing with flour in it
- No fruits, too
- No whole grains either
- Proteins up to 6 ounces per day, only lean sources though
- Have 4 to 5 servings of lentils or beans per week

Healthy fats should be included, too. This includes fats from plant sources like seeds and nuts. Fruits rich in healthy monounsaturated fats are also good choices. This includes avocados, which is also rich in beta carotene, lutein, and vitamin E. These are potent antioxidants that can further improve your health status. These can also help you burn those pesky excess fats around your belly faster.

Other good plant sources of healthy fats include olive oil, nut oils, and canola oil. These will be mainstays in your dressing recipes for your salads, especially during Phase 1. These will also be your oil of choice when you sauté or fry (yes, fry) lean meats such as pan-seared salmon or pan-grilled chicken breasts.

Fatty fishes such as mackerel and salmon are also great sources.

DASH for weight loss Phase 2

After the 14-day Phase 1, the same food list will be used for the next phase. Other healthy food will also be reintroduced into your diet. That means you will be able to eat healthy starches at this point. Some fruits and a few sweet treats are allowed now, too.

Your new food list, which you will follow from now on, will be:

- Whole grains at 6 to 8 servings per day. Choices include breads and pasta made from whole grain is best. Whole grain cereals are also part of your choices.
- Fruits, as mentioned, are now OK. You can have them fresh or frozen. Your daily servings of fruit should be around 4 to 5. Low sugar fruits and those rich in nutrients are great choices. Examples are berries and avocados.
- Dairy would best be limited to yogurt or low fat milk. Daily servings are 2 to 3, just like in Phase 1.
- Sugars are also now allowed, but should be limited. Stay away from unhealthy sweets such as those that contain white or refined sugar. You are limited to 3 to 4 servings per week only. That means a small serving of frozen yogurt instead of regular ice cream, a bite or two of cake or pie, or a tablespoon or two of custard. You can enjoy some of the old sweets you used to have but in smaller quantities. It is better to make healthier substitutions, too. For example, instead of regular chocolate cake, choose one that uses dark (75% cocoa or more) chocolate. Instead of regular snack bars, choose

granola. Instead of regular chocolate candy, choses dark chocolate bar.

- Alcohol can be included in the diet, but those who are not taking alcohol on a regular basis are better off without it. A glass of wine is equivalent to 1 fruit serving. You can substitute the small amount of wine for your daily fruit serving.

CHAPTER 2

DASH FOOD GROUPS AND RECOMMENDED SERVINGS

The diet teaches you to eat certain healthy food groups in certain amounts. These were based on studies and recommendations designed to ensure that you are getting the right amount of nutrients from the right sources. You should also aim to get all the daily servings recommended to gain a healthier body and a slimmer waistline in no time.

Grains & products with grain

Daily servings: 7–8

Serving sizes:

- 1/2 cup cereal, pasta, or rice, cooked
- 1 oz. dry cereal
- 1 bread slice

Examples:

- pita bread
- whole wheat bread
- crackers
- English muffin
- bagel

- grits
- cereals
- oatmeal
- popcorn
- unsalted pretzels

Vegetables

Daily servings: 4–5

Serving sizes:

- 6 oz. vegetable juice
- 1 cup raw leafy vegetable
- 1/2 cup vegetable, cooked

Examples:

- Broccoli
- Tomatoes
- Squash
- Carrots
- Sweet potatoes
- Potatoes
- Green peas
- Lima beans
- Green beans
- Collards
- Spinach
- Turnip greens
- Kale

- Artichokes

Fruits

Daily servings: 4–5

Serving sizes:

- 1/4 cup dried fruit
- 1 medium fruit
- 1/2 cup canned, fresh or frozen fruit
- 6 oz. fruit juice

Examples

- Apricots
- Dates
- Raisins
- Prunes
- Bananas
- Strawberries
- Grapes
- Oranges
- Grapefruit
- Tangerines
- Orange juice
- Grapefruit juice
- Melons
- Mangoes
- Pineapples
- Peaches

Fat-free or Low-fat dairy

Daily servings: 2–3

Serving sizes:

- 1 cup yogurt
- 8 oz. milk
- 1 1/2 oz. cheese

Examples:

- low-fat (1%) or fat free (skim) milk
- low-fat or fat free regular or frozen yogurt
- low-fat or fat free buttermilk
- fat-free and low-fat cheese

Meats, fish and poultry

Daily servings: not more than 2

Serving sizes:

- 3 oz. cooked poultry, fish, or meats

Examples:

- only lean meats
- remove any visible fats
- remove skin poultry
- broil, boil, or roast instead of frying

Dry beans, nuts, and seeds

Daily servings: 4 to 5 a week

Serving sizes:

- 2 tablespoons (1/2 oz.) seeds
- 1/3 cup (1 1/2 oz.) nuts
- 1/2 cup cooked dry beans

Examples:

- Almonds
- Mixed nuts
- Walnuts
- Peanuts
- Sunflower seed
- Lentils
- Kidney beans
- Peas
- Filberts

Oils & fats

Daily servings: 2–3

Serving sizes:

- 1 teaspoon soft margarine
- 1 teaspoon vegetable oil
- 1 tablespoon low-fat mayonnaise
- 2 tablespoon light salad dressing

Examples:

- low-fat mayonnaise
- soft margarine
- vegetable oil (such as corn, safflower, olive, or canola)
- light salad dressing

Sweets

Weekly servings: 5 in a week

Serving sizes:

- 1/2 oz. jelly beans
- 1 tablespoon sugar
- 8 oz. lemonade
- 1 tablespoon jelly or jam

Examples:

- Sugar
- Maple syrup
- Jam
- Jelly
- Gelatin, in fruit flavors
- Hard candy
- Jelly beans
- Fruit punch
- Ices Sorbet

CHAPTER 3

BREAKFAST DASH RECIPES

Edamame Hummus Wrap

4 servings

Ingredients

- 2¼ cups shelled frozen edamame, thawed before using
- 3 tablespoons extra-virgin olive oil, divided
- 4 tablespoons fresh squeezed lemon juice, divided
- 2 tablespoons tahini
- ¾ teaspoon ground pepper, divided
- ½ teaspoon ground cumin
- ½ teaspoon salt
- 1 large garlic clove, chopped
- ¼ cup sliced fresh parsley
- 2 cups very thin slices of green cabbage
- 1 scallion, sliced thinly
- ½ cup sliced orange bell pepper
- 4 pieces 8- to 9-inch whole-wheat or spinach tortillas

Make

1. Put edamame with 2 tablespoons oil, 3 tablespoons lemon juice, cumin, garlic, tahini, salt and ½ teaspoon pepper in a food processor. Pulse until it turns into a smooth mixture.

2. Put the remaining ¼ teaspoon pepper, 1 tablespoon oil and 1 tablespoon lemon juice in a medium-sized bowl. Whisk well. Put bell peppers, cabbage, parsley and scallions into the bow with the dressing. Toss until everything is coated evenly with the dressing.

3. Scoop out ½ cup of edamame hummus and spread over the lower third of a tortilla. Top the hummus with ½ cup of cabbage mixture. Carefully roll the tortilla tightly.

4. Slice in half before serving.

Nutrition information

Per serving size: 1 wrap

- 339 calories
- 35 g carbohydrates
- 8 g fiber
- 0 g added sugars
- 4 g sugars
- 20 g fat(3 g sat)
- 0 mg cholesterol
- 14 g protein
- 307 mcg folate
- 54 mg vitamin C
- 1,320 IU vitamin A
- 4 mg iron
- 104 mg calcium
- 641 mg potassium
- 480 mg sodium

Black Bean & Salmon Tostadas

4 servings

Ingredients

- Canola oil cooking spray
- 8 pieces 6-inch corn tortillas
- 1 6- to 7-ounce can skinless, boneless wild Alaskan salmon, liquid drained
- 2 tablespoons minced pickled jalapeños
- 2 tablespoons pickling juice from the pickled jalapeno jar, divided
- 1 medium avocado, diced
- 2 cups shredded cabbage or coleslaw mix
- 1 15-ounce can black beans, drained and rinsed
- 2 tablespoons chopped cilantro
- 3 tablespoons reduced-fat sour cream
- 2 scallions, chopped
- 2 tablespoons prepared salsa
- Lime wedges

Make

1. Put oven racks in the lower and upper third positions. Prepare oven temperature to 375F. Spray both sides of each tortilla lightly with some cooking spray.

2. Arrange the tortilla on 2 cookie or baking sheets. Bake tortilla in the oven, turning once for even cooking. Bake until both sides are lightly browned, about 12 to 4 minutes.

3. Put avocado, jalapeno and salon in a bowl. Toss to mix. Get another bowl. Put pickling juice, cilantro and cabbage. Mix and set aside.

4. Put sour cream, scallions, salsa and black beans in a food processor. Pulse until mixture becomes smooth. Transfer the black bean mixture into a microwave-safe bowl. Heat on high for 2 minutes until hot. Alternatively, transfer into a saucepan and put over high heat until mixture is hot. Stir to keep the bottom of the mixture from burning.

5. Place one tortilla on a plate or chopping board. Spread some of the bean mixture over each tortilla. Top with some of the salmon mixture. Add some of the cabbage salad on top.

6. Roll up or fold the tortilla in two. Serve with lime wedges.

Nutrition information

Per serving size: 2 tostadas

- 406 calories
- 45 g carbohydrates
- 12 g fiber
- 0 g added sugars
- 6 g sugars
- 17 g protein
- 19 g fat (3 g saturated fat)
- 16 mg cholesterol
- 107 mcg folate

- 35 mg vitamin C
- 622 IU vitamin A
- 3 mg iron
- 116 mg calcium
- 679 mg potassium
- 392 mg sodium

Black Bean and Zucchini Tacos with Avocado Crema

4 servings

Ingredients

<u>For the tacos</u>

- 1 large zucchini, grated
- 1 15-ounce can black beans, drained and rinsed
- 1/4 teaspoon garlic powder
- 1/2 teaspoon chipotle powder
- 1/4 teaspoon paprika
- 1/2 teaspoon chili powder
- 8 corn tortillas

<u>For the salsa</u>

- 1 1/2 cups diced tomatoes
- Juice of 1 lime
- 1/2 cup red onion
- 1/4 teaspoon salt

<u>For the avocado crema</u>

- 1 avocado, remove pit
- Juice from 1 lime
- 1/2 cup low-fat Greek yogurt
- 1/4 teaspoon salt

Make

1. Mix the ingredients for the salsa in a small bowl. Set aside.

2. Remove the avocado flesh and put in a food processor. Add salt, lime juice and yogurt. Pulse until and well combined. Transfer into a small bowl and set aside.

3. Mix spices, black beans and zucchini in a bowl. Stir to mix.

4. Heat the tortillas, over a stove or in a microwave.

5. Divide the zucchini-black bean mixture between the tortillas. Spoon salsa over the bean mixture. Top with some of the avocado crema.

6. Roll the tortilla or fold in half. Serve with more salsa and crema on the side, if desired.

Nutrition Information

Per serving size: 1 taco

- 245 calories
- 35 g carbohydrates
- 5 g sugar
- 9 g fiber
- 10 g fat (2 g saturated fat)
- 9 g proteins

Open-Face Tuna Salad

2 servings

Ingredients

- 1 5-ounce can low-sodium tuna packed in water, drained
- 2 tablespoons freshly squeezed lemon juice
- 2 tablespoons extra-virgin olive oil
- 2 tablespoons chopped fresh parsley
- 2 green onions, sliced
- Black pepper
- 2 slices multigrain bread
- 1/3 cup halved cherry tomatoes
- 1/3 cup fresh arugula
- 1/4 cup reduced-fat whipped cream cheese

Make

1. Combine lemon juice, green onion, pepper, parsley and oil in a bowl.

2. Put tuna in a separate bowl. Pour about 2/3 of oil-juice mixture over the tune. Reserve the remaining mixture. Mix tuna and oil-juice mixture well.

3. Coat both sides of the bread lightly with the reserved oil-juice mixture. Toast the bread until golden on both sides. Set aside.

4. Pour any remaining oil-juice mixture over the arugula. Toss to mix. Spoon about 2 tablespoons cream cheese over each

toast. Spread evenly over one side of the bread. Spoon half of the tuna mixture over each bread slice. Arrange half of the arugula then half of the cherry tomatoes over the tuna.

5. Serve.

Nutrition Information

Per serving size: 1 open-face sandwich

- 361 calories
- 18 g carbohydrates
- 5 g sugar
- 5 g fiber
- 22 g fat (6 g saturated fat)
- 24 g proteins

Toast with Banana, Chia Seed & Sun Butter

1 serving

Ingredients

- 1 slice 100% whole wheat bread
- 1/2 medium banana, *sliced*
- 1 tablespoon sun butter (sunflower butter)
- 1/2 teaspoon chia seeds

Make

1. Spread sunbutter over the bread.

2. Arrange banana slices over the sunbutter.

3. Sprinkle with chia seeds.

4. Serve.

Nutritional Information

Per serving size: 1 toast

- 209.9 calories
- 27.6 g carbohydrates
- 9.7 g sugar
- 5.1 g fiber
- 9.6 g fat
- 8.5 g protein
- 175.8 mg sodium

Savory Oatmeal with Cheddar & Fried Egg

1 serving

Ingredients

- 3/4 cup water
- 1/4 cup dry quick-cooking steel cut oats
- salt and pepper
- 1 teaspoon coconut oil, divided
- 2 tablespoons shredded white cheddar cheese
- 2 tablespoons finely sliced onions
- 1/4 cup diced red peppers
- 1 large egg

Optional toppings

- sliced green onions
- chopped walnuts

Make

1. Boil water in a saucepan then add the oatmeal. Reduce heat slightly and cook oatmeal for 3 minutes. Remove the heat once oatmeal is tender and all the water has been absorbed. Add cheese into the saucepan and stir to mix. Season with some pepper and salt. Transfer into a serving bowl.

2. Place a non-stick pan over medium-high heat. Add ½ teaspoon coconut oil. Once oil is heated, add the vegetables.

Cook the vegetables until softened, about 2 to 3 minutes. Spoon cooked vegetables over the oats.

3. Pour the remaining oil into the same pan. Fry the eggs. Transfer cooked eggs over the vegetables.

4. Serve.

Nutrition Information

Per serving size: 1 bowl

- 262 calories
- 18 g total carbohydrate
- 3 g sugar
- 3 g dietary fiber
- 16 g total fat (9 g saturated fat)
- 201 mg cholesterol
- 178 mg sodium
- 13 g protein

Eggplant Bowl with Cilantro and Mint Chutney

4 servings

Ingredients

Eggplant & red pepper sauce

- 1 1/2 pounds eggplant, sliced into 1/4-inch rounds
- 1 tablespoon olive oil
- non-stick cooking spray
- 1 large red pepper, seeds discarded, diced finely
- 2 garlic cloves, minced
- 1 green onion (only light green and white parts), chopped roughly
- 1 medium red onion, chopped finely
- 2/3 cup canned diced tomatoes
- 2 tablespoons tomato paste
- 1/4 teaspoon ground cumin
- 1 teaspoon paprika
- pepper and salt, to taste

Cilantro and mint chutney

- 1/2 cup cilantro leaves and tender stems
- 1/2 cup fresh mint leaves
- 1 green onion (only dark green part), chopped roughly
- 1 garlic clove, chopped roughly
- 1/2-inch piece fresh ginger, peel then slice
- 2 teaspoons agave (or any type of sweetener)

- 1 tablespoon apple cider vinegar
- 1/8 to 1/4 teaspoon salt

For serving

- 1 14-ounce can garbanzo beans, drained then rinsed
- 4 cups cooked basmati rice
- 1/2 cup low-fat yogurt

Make

1. Preheat the broiler.

2. Arrange eggplant rounds on a paper towel. Sprinkle the eggplant with some salt. Set aside and let the salt draw out water from the eggplant. Wipe down any moisture from the eggplant. Get a baking sheet and line it foil. Spray the surface of the foil lightly with some cooking spray. Arrange eggplant slices on the lined baking sheet in a single layer. Broil the eggplant slices for 4 to 5 minutes on each side. Once done, pile the eggplant slices on a foil and wrap. Leave to rest for a few minutes. Open the foil packet and separate the peel from the eggplant slices. Set aside on a bowl.

3. Pour 1 tablespoon olive oil in a large sauté pan. Add red onions and cook until softened. Stir constantly to keep the onions from burning. Add the red pepper and garlic. Continue cooking for 5 minutes. Increase heat to medium.

4. Add the eggplant flesh, diced tomatoes, cumin, paprika, pepper, salt, tomato paste ad green onions. Cook for 2 more minutes then remove from heat. Adjust the seasonings according to taste. Transfer the mixture in a food processor and blend. An immersion blender may be used instead, if available.

5. Place all the ingredients for the chutney in a food processor. Process until it becomes a smooth mixture. Add water tablespoon by tablespoon to adjust the consistency.

6. Divide the cooked rice between 4 serving bowls. Top with garbanzos. Spoon some of the eggplant mixture over the rice-bean bowl. Spoon some chutney.

7. Serve topped with the yogurt.

Nutrition Information

Per serving size: 1 bowl

- 458 calories
- 86.5 g total carbohydrate
- 17 g sugar
- 14.5 g dietary fiber
- 7.2 g total fat (1.3 g saturated fat)
- 1.9 mg cholesterol
- 439 mg sodium
- 15 g protein

Breakfast Fruit Parfait

4 servings

Ingredients

- 4 cups mixed strawberries and blueberries
- 5 1/3 cups light fat-free vanilla yogurt
- 1 cup granola, crumbled

Make

1. Place 2/3 cup of yogurt into each of the 4 juice or parfait glasses.

2. Add a layer of ½ cup berries then 2 tablespoons of granola.

3. Add another 2/3 cup of yogurt, then half a cup of the berries and then 2 tablespoons of crumbled granola.

4. Chill or serve immediately.

Nutrition Information

Per serving size: 1 parfait

- 245 calories
- 49 g carbohydrate
- 27 g sugars
- 6 g dietary fiber
- 4.0 g fat (1.4 g saturated fat)
- 5 mg cholesterol
- 90 mg sodium
- 8 g protein
- 520 mg potassium

CHAPTER 4

LUNCH DASH RECIPES

Stuffed Roasted Squash

4 servings

Ingredients

- 2 small delicata squash, sliced in half, seeds removed
- ½ teaspoon salt, divided
- 6 teaspoons extra-virgin olive oil, divided
- 1 cup water
- ½ cup bulgur
- 1 ½ cups (around 250 g or 8 oz.) lean ground beef
- 1 small onion, chopped
- ½ cup plain yogurt, low-fat or nonfat
- 2 tablespoons chili powder
- 4 teaspoons toasted pepitas

Make

1. Prepare oven heat to 425F. Use 2 teaspoons oil for brushing the cut side of each half of the squash. Sprinkle ¼ teaspoon of salt over all the squash, over the oiled sides. Arrange the squash on a baking or cookie sheet, face down. Bake the squash in the preheated oven until browned and tender, about

25 to 30 minutes of baking. Remove squash once done and set aside.

2. Pour water into a small saucepan. Add the bulger. Set the saucepan over high heat until boiling. Lower setting to a simmer. Cover the saucepan and cook until the bulgur becomes tender, around 10 minutes of simmering. Drain any liquid that remains. Set aside.

3. Place a large skillet on a stove over medium heat. Pour the remaining 4 teaspoons of oil into the skillet. Put the onions as well. Cook until it starts to turn brown. Add chili powder, remaining ¼ teaspoon salt and beef. Cook while breaking up the meat for faster and even cooking. Once beef is done, no longer pink and no more liquid in the skillet, add the bulgur. Cook for another minute and turn off the heat. Add yogurt and stir in well.

4. Spoon ¾ cup of this mixture into each of the squash halves. Sprinkle with pepitas.

5. Serve while still warm.

Nutrition Information

Per serving size: ½ stuffed squash

- 318 calories
- 35 g carbohydrates
- 0 g added sugars

- 6 g sugars
- 9 g fiber
- 14 g fat (3 g saturated fat)
- 37 mg cholesterol
- 45 mcg folate
- 18 g protein
- 480 mg sodium
- 23 mg vitamin C
- 17,338 IU vitamin A
- 153 mg calcium
- 841 mg potassium
- 3 mg iron

Roasted Chicken, Potatoes, and Brussels Sprouts

4 servings

Ingredients

- 1 pound skinless boneless chicken breasts, sliced into 4 pieces
- 3 cups red or Yukon gold potatoes, sliced into bite-size pieces
- 4 cups quartered trimmed Brussels sprouts
- 1 cup diced onions
- 1/3 cup vinaigrette dressing
- 2 teaspoons Dijon mustard
- Juice of 1 medium-sized lemon
- 1 1/2 teaspoons oregano
- 1/4 cup quartered Kalamata olives
- 1/4 teaspoon garlic salt
- Freshly ground black pepper

Make

1. Prepare oven temperature to 400F.

2. Arrange chicken pieces in a single layer in the center of a sheet baking pan. Arrange the Brussels sprouts on one side of the pan. Arrange the potatoes on the other side. Arrange the onions in any available space.

3. Whisk garlic salt, oregano, mustard, lemon juice and vinaigrette in a small bowl. Drizzle the vinaigrette-mustard mixture over the chicken and vegetables on the sheet

pan. Sprinkle pepper and olives all over the chicken and vegetables. Bake everything in the preheated oven until the chicken is done all the way through. Transfer and divide the cooked chicken on serving plates.

4. Stir the vegetables to mix. Return the sheet pan with the vegetables into the oven. Continue roasting until the potatoes are tender when pierced with a fork and the Brussels sprouts are crispy.

5. Divide the roasted vegetables among the serving plates.

6. Serve while still warm.

Nutrition Information

Per serving:

- 361 calories
- 37 g carbohydrates
- 7 g fiber
- 10 g fat (2 g saturated fat)
- 32 g protein

Salmon with Asparagus & Farro

4 servings

Ingredients

- ¾ cup farro
- 3 cups water
- 1 tablespoon extra-virgin olive oil
- 1 bunch trimmed asparagus, sliced into 1-inch pieces
- 2 cups leeks, light green and white parts only, sliced in half and sliced thinly
- 2 garlic cloves, minced
- 3 tablespoons white miso
- 2 cups low-sodium chicken broth
- 1¼ pounds skinned wild Alaskan salmon fillet, sliced into 1-inch pieces
- ¼ teaspoon pepper
- 3 tablespoons minced fresh basil

Make

1. Put water and farro in a saucepan. Set over a stove on high heat and allow to boil. Lower heat setting to medium low. Cover the saucepan and let the farro cook for 30 minutes until it becomes soft yet still chewy. Remove from heat and drain any water that remains. Set the farro aside.

2. Put oil into a large saucepan and heat over medium setting while the farro is still cooking. Sauté the leeks for 2 minutes until it soften. Add garlic and asparagus and cook. Stir

constantly until the asparagus turns bright green in color. Add miso and broth into the saucepan. Raise the heat setting to high and allow the liquid to boil. Once boiling, add salmon. Reduce heat setting down to a simmer and cook for 3 minutes. Turn off the heat. Add pepper and basil. Stir gently to mix.

3. Scoop the farro between 4 deep serving bowls. Carefully ladle the soup into each bowl. Top each bowl with salmon pieces.

4. Serve.

Nutrition information

Per serving size: ½ cup farro & 1½ cups stew

- 407 calories
- 40 g carbohydrates
- 5 g fiber
- 0 g added sugars
- 4 g sugars
- 11 g fat (2 g saturated fat)
- 66 mg cholesterol
- 37 g protein
- 432 mg sodium
- 129 mcg folate
- 12 mg vitamin C
- 1,613 IU vitamin A
- 3 mg iron
- 125 mg calcium
- 847 mg potassium

Chicken and African Sweet Potato Stew

4 servings

Ingredients

- 1 pound skinless, boneless chicken thighs, sliced into bite-sized pieces
- ¾ teaspoon salt, divided
- 2 teaspoons ground coriander, divided
- 2 tablespoons extra-virgin olive oil, divided
- 1 tablespoon grated fresh ginger
- 1 large onion, halved then sliced
- 1 large sweet potato, peeled then cubed
- ¼ cup natural smooth peanut butter
- 1 28-ounce can no-salt-added whole tomatoes, chopped, reserve the juice
- ¼ teaspoon cayenne pepper
- 2 tablespoons lime juice, divided
- 1 cup whole-wheat couscous
- 1½ cups water
- 1 cup chopped cilantro

Make

1. Mix ½ teaspoon salt, coriander and chicken pieces.

2. Pour oil in a large skillet and heat over medium-high setting. Once hot, add chicken. Stir and cook until all sides are browned. Transfer cooked chicken to a plate and set aside.

3. Pour the remaining oil into the same skillet. Sauté ginger and onion for 3 to 5 minutes until these turn light brown. Add reserved juice from the canned tomato, 1 tablespoon of the lime juice, ¼ teaspoon salt, remaining 1 teaspoon coriander, cayenne, peanut butter, tomatoes and sweet potato. Allow the mixture to boil then lower heat down to a simmer. Cover the skillet and cook until the sweet potatoes become tender. Stir occasionally. Put the chicken into the skillet and any juices that accumulated. Continue cooking until the chicken is heated through. This will take about 2 minutes.

4. Pour water in a separate saucepan while the stew is cooking. Once the water is boiling, add the couscous. Stir in the remaining 1 tablespoon of fresh lime juice. Cover the saucepan and remove from heat. Set aside the couscous aside to cook with the residual heat inside the saucepan, for about 5 minutes. Once couscous is ready, use a fork to fluff it. Add the cilantro into the couscous and stir.

5. Spoon couscous into serving bowls. Ladle the stew over the couscous ad serve while still warm.

Nutrition Information

Per serving size: 1 cup couscous & 1¾ cups stew

- 615 calories
- 66 g carbohydrates
- 0 g added sugars

- 12 g sugars
- 13 g fiber
- 24 g fat (5 g saturated fats)
- 76 mg cholesterol
- 35 g protein
- 457 mg sodium
- 14,508 IU vitamin A
- 37 mcg folate
- 45 mg vitamin C
- 5 mg iron
- 142 mg calcium
- 954 mg potassium

Apple & Parsnip Curry Soup

4 servings

Ingredients

- 5 medium peeled parsnips, cored then chopped
- 1 tablespoon extra-virgin olive oil
- 3 garlic cloves, chopped finely
- 1 onion, chopped finely
- 1 cup water
- 1 large peeled Granny Smith apple, cubed
- 4 cups chicken broth, low-sodium
- 1 peeled medium russet potato, chopped
- 1½ teaspoons curry powder, mild, if desired
- 1 teaspoon ground cumin
- 1½ teaspoons ground coriander, add more as garnish
- 4 teaspoons lemon juice
- ½ teaspoon ground ginger
- ¼ teaspoon fresh ground pepper
- ½ teaspoon salt
- ½ cup plain low-fat yogurt

Make

1. Pour oil into a large pot. Place on a stove set over medium high heat. Sauté onion and parsnips for about 5 to 7 minutes until onions start to turn brown. Put the garlic into the pot and continue cooking for 45 seconds until it becomes fragrant. Add apple, potato, water, broth, ginger, cumin and coriander. Let the

stew boil then cover. Lower the heat down to a simmer. Cook the vegetables until tender. This takes about 20 minutes.

2. Puree the soup with immersion blender. A blender or food processor may be used to puree the soup in batches. Take precautions when handling the hot soup. Once pureed, stir in pepper, salt and lemon juice.

3. Ladle into serving bowls. Add a dollop of yogurt and garnish with coriander. Serve while still warm.

Nutrition information

Per serving size: 2 cups

- 303 calories
- 58 g carbohydrates
- 0 g added sugars
- 19 g sugars
- 12 g fiber
- 6 g fat (1 g saturated fat)
- 6 mg cholesterol
- 8 g protein
- 132 mcg folate
- 444 mg sodium
- 41 mg vitamin C
- 52 IU vitamin A
- 2 mg iron
- 152 mg calcium
- 1,202 mg potassium

Spaghetti Squash & Seared Chicken with Mango Salsa

4 servings

Ingredients

- 1 peeled ripe mango, diced
- ½ cup red onion, diced finely
- 1 fresh jalapeño, minced
- ¼ cup fresh cilantro, chopped
- 1 tablespoon light brown sugar
- 2 tablespoons red-wine vinegar
- 1¼ teaspoons salt, divided
- 2 8-ounce skinless, boneless chicken breasts, halved
- 1 spaghetti squash, sliced in half lengthwise, seeds removed
- ¼ cup toasted sliced almonds
- 2 tablespoons canola oil or coconut oil, divided

Make

1. Put brown sugar, ¾ teaspoon salt, vinegar, cilantro, onion, jalapeno and mango in a bowl. Stir to combine.

2. Arrange the squash on a baking dish with the cut side down. Put 2 tablespoons of water into the baking dish. Bake in a preheated 350F oven until the squash softens. This takes around 10 to 14 minutes.

3. Get a meat mallet and pound the chicken until the thickness is even all over at ½ inch thick. Sprinkle all sides of the chicken with ½ teaspoon salt.

4. Pour 1 tablespoon oil into a large skillet set over medium high heat. Once oil and skillet are hot, put the chicken in. cook until the internal temperature reaches 165F. Cook on both sides for about 3 to 5 minutes.

5. Remove the squash once done. Cool slightly. Scrape off the flesh of the squash from its shell. Place the flesh in a medium bowl. Put ¼ teaspoon salt and the remaining 1 tablespoon oil with the squash. Mix well.

6. Place cooked chicken on a serving plate. Spoon some of the squash beside the chicken. Spoon some salsa on the side of the chicken. Sprinkle everything with almonds and serve.

Nutrition information

Per serving size: 3 oz. chicken, ½ cup salsa & 1 cup squash

- 366 calories
- 38 g carbohydrates
- 7 g fiber
- 3 g added sugars
- 23 g sugars
- 13 g fat (7 g saturated fat)
- 63 mg cholesterol

- 27 g protein
- 461 mg sodium
- 1,348 IU vitamin A
- 70 mcg folate
- 47 mg vitamin C
- 2 mg iron
- 106 mg calcium
- 761 mg potassium

Edamame and Quinoa Indian Burger

4 servings

Ingredients

- 1 cup water
- ½ cup quinoa
- 1½ cups frozen edamame, thaw before using
- 1 large egg
- 3 scallions, sliced, divided
- 1 tablespoon minced fresh ginger
- ½ teaspoon plus ⅛ teaspoon salt, divided
- 1¼ teaspoons garam masala
- ¼ teaspoon cayenne pepper
- ¾ cup plain low-fat yogurt
- 2 tablespoons extra-virgin olive oil, divided
- ½ cup chopped English cucumber
- ¼ teaspoon ground pepper
- ¼ cup chopped fresh cilantro
- 1 large tomato, sliced thickly into 4

Make

1. Place water and quinoa in a saucepan. Place over a stove and let the water boil. Lower the heat and cover the saucepan. Let the water simmer until all is absorbed by the quinoa. This takes around 15 minutes. Turn the heat off and let the

quinoa stand for 5 minutes. Fluff the quinoa and put into a food processor. Add 2 scallions (chopped), ginger, cayenne, garam masala, egg, and edamame. Season with ½ teaspoon salt. Pulse until everything forms a smooth mixture. Transfer into a shallow dish. Divide the mixture into four. Form each section into patties, about 3 ½ inches round.

2. Heat a large noon-stick skillet on a stove set to medium high heat. Add 1 tablespoon oil. Swirl the skillet to coat the sides with oil. Add the patties and cook until browned. Flip and brown the other side.

3. While the patties are cooking, prepare the yogurt sauce. Get a mixing bowl. Put cilantro, remaining chopped scallion, 1/8 teaspoon salt, pepper, cucumber and yogurt. Stir to mix well.

4. Place cooked patties on a serving plate. Top with a slice of tomato.

5. Pour about ¼ cup of the yogurt sauce over the burgers. Serve.

Nutrition information

Per serving size: 1 burger, ¼ cup sauce & 1 tomato slice

- 285 calories
- 29 g carbohydrates
- 6 g fiber
- 0 g added sugars
- 9 g sugars

- 13 g fat (2 g saturated fat)
- 49 mg cholesterol
- 14 g protein
- 427 mg sodium
- 1,439 IU vitamin A
- 252 mcg folate
- 22 mg vitamin C
- 3 mg iron
- 161 mg calcium
- 822 mg potassium

CHAPTER 5

DINNER DASH RECIPES

Farro and Roasted Vegetable Salad

15 servings

Ingredients

- 3 cups dry farro
- 3 cups broccoli florets
- 3 cups cauliflower florets
- 2 tablespoons extra virgin olive oil
- 2 peeled onions, sliced into wedges
- 1/4 teaspoon freshly ground black pepper
- 1/4 teaspoon salt
- 3 tablespoons chopped fresh parsley
- 1 cup dried cranberries
- 1 cup chopped hazelnuts
- Juice of 2 lemons (about 1/4 cup)
- Zest of 2 lemons
- 1/4 cup apple cider vinegar
- 1/2 cup extra-virgin olive oil
- 1/2 teaspoon salt

Make

1. Put farro inside a large pot. Pour water enough to cover the farro with about 2 inches of water. Bring the farro to a boil over high heat then lower down to a simmer. Cook until farro becomes tender, about 30 minutes of simmering. Drain any excess water. Set farro aside and allow to cool.

2. Prepare the oven temperature to 450F. Put onion wedges, broccoli and cauliflower in a salad bowl. Drizzle with the olive oil and season with pepper and salt. Toss to mix well. Arrange the vegetables in a single layer on a baking sheet. Roast in the preheated oven until caramelized. This will take around 20 to 25 minutes. Remove roasted vegetables from the oven and allow to cool.

3. Juice the two lemons and put in a measuring cup. Add the zest as well. Pour enough apple cider vinegar into the measuring cup to bring the measurement to a total of ½ cup. Add some salt to season the vinaigrette. Pour into a bowl and add ½ cup of olive oil. Whisk well to mix.

4. Mix cooled roasted vegetables and farro in a large salad bowl. Add parsley, cranberries and hazelnuts. Drizzle the vinaigrette over everything. Gently toss to coat everything evenly.

5. Serve at room temperature or chilled.

Nutrition information

Per serving size: 1 cup of salad

- 322 calories
- 7 g sugar
- 6 g fiber
- 16 g fat (2 g saturated fat)
- 9 g protein
- 137 mg sodium

Salmon Edamame Cakes

4 servings

Ingredients

- 2 cups flaked cooked salmon
- 1/4 cup panko
- 2 large egg whites
- 1 tablespoon minced fresh peeled ginger
- 1 scallion, only the green and white parts, chopped finely
- 1 tablespoon minced fresh cilantro
- 1 garlic clove, crushed
- 1/2 cup thawed frozen edamame
- Canola oil
- Lime wedges, for serving

Make

1. Put panko, salmon, ginger, cilantro, garlic, scallion and egg whites in a medium-sized bowl. Mix.

2. Ad edamame and mix well.

3. Divide the mixture into 4. Make each section into 3 ½-inch cakes.

4. Place cakes on a plate lined with wax paper. Chill the cakes for 15 to 30 minutes.

5. Heat oil in a large skillet set over medium heat.

6. Once hot, cook the cakes until the bottom starts to turn brown, about 3 to 4 minutes. Flip and cook the other side as well.

7. Transfer to a plate and serve while still hot. Serve with some lime wedges.

Nutrition information

Per serving size: 1 cake

- 267 calories
- 1 g fiber
- 1 g fat
- 21 g protein
- 166 mg sodium

Spiced North African Turkey with Avocado-Grapefruit Relish

6 servings

Ingredients

- 1 peeled avocado, pitted, flesh diced
- 3 seedless large grapefruit
- ¼ cup thin red onion slices
- 1 tablespoon fresh chopped mint
- 2 tablespoons fresh chopped cilantro
- 1 tablespoon honey
- 1 tablespoon red-wine vinegar
- ½ teaspoon ground cloves
- ½ teaspoon ground cinnamon
- ½ teaspoon ground allspice
- ¼ cup mild chili powder
- ¼ teaspoon salt
- 2 teaspoons canola oil
- 1½ pounds (about ¼ inch thick)turkey cutlets

Make

1. Heat the oven to temperature of 400F.

2. Peel the grapefruit and remove the white pit. Separate the sections and remove the membrane. Place grapefruit flesh into a bowl. Add cilantro, onions, honey, vinegar, mint and avocados. Toss gently to mix. Set aside.

3. Mix salt, cinnamon, allspice, cloves and chili powder in a shallow dish. Put turkey slices into the spice mixture and dredge on all sides. Shake off excess spice mix and place coated turkey slices on a plate.

4. Heat an oven-proof skillet on a stove over medium high heat. Add oil. Once hot, cook the cutlets. Once the outside of the cutlets turn brown, flip and remove the skillet from the stove. Place the skillet in the preheated oven. Bake until the center of the turkey slices are no longer pink. Bake for about 4 to 6 minutes.

5. Transfer cooked turkey slices on a serving plate. Serve with the grapefruit-avocado relish.

Nutrition information

Per serving size: about 1 cup or so

- 270 calories
- 23 g carbohydrates
- 6 g fiber
- 3 g added sugars
- 15 g sugars
- 8 g fat (1 g saturated fat)
- 45 mg cholesterol
- 31 g protein
- 355 mg sodium

- 3,251 IU vitamin A
- 47 mcg folate
- 61 mg vitamin C
- 3 mg iron
- 49 mg calcium
- 515 mg potassium

Dan Dan Noodles with Baby Bok Choy & Chicken

6 servings

Ingredients

- 1 large trimmed, skinless, boneless chicken breast
- 3 tablespoons fresh chopped ginger, divided
- 1¼ cups low-sodium chicken broth, divided
- 2 teaspoons hot chili oil
- 2 tablespoons reduced-sodium soy sauce
- ¼ cup natural peanut butter
- 1 tablespoon Chinese black vinegar
- ¼ teaspoon sugar
- 3 tablespoons canola oil or peanut oil, divided
- 12 ounces linguine or Chinese flat noodles
- 3 scallions, chopped coarsely
- 1 pound halved baby bok choy
- 2 tablespoons chopped garlic
- 2 teaspoons toasted sesame oil
- ¼ teaspoon crushed red pepper
- 2 tablespoons toasted sesame seeds

Make

1. Put chicken, 1 tablespoon of the chopped ginger and 1 cup of the broth in a saucepan. Place on a stove with heat on medium high setting. When the broth starts to simmer, cover the saucepan and lower the heat.

2. Cook the chicken until the thickest center part reaches a temperature of 165F. Turn the chicken 1 to 2 times to cook evenly. This takes around 15 minutes. Place the chicken on a clean chopping board. Set aside the liquid used for poaching the chicken. When chicken is no longer too hot to work with, shred and put in a bowl. Set aside.

3. Add the rest of the ¼ cup of broth into the saucepan with the poaching liquid. Add the chili oil, vinegar, sugar, soy sauce and peanut butter. Whisk well and set aside.

4.   Boil water in a pot and follow the cooking directions for the noodles or pasta found on the package. Drain once cooked and then rinse with cold running water.

5. Heat a skillet. Add oil. Swirl to grease the sides of the skillet. Once skillet and oil are hot, add crushed red pepper, garlic and 2 tablespoons ginger. Sauté until fragrant but do not allow the spices to brown. Transfer immediately into the saucepan with the peanut butter mix. Let the sauce simmer then remove from heat.

6. In the same skillet where the spices were sautéed, add 1 ½ tablespoons canola or peanut oil. Swirl to coat the sides. Once hot, add the bok choy into the skillet. Stir while cooking until bok choy becomes crisp-tender. Turn off the heat. Put noodles into the skillet with the bok choy. Toss to mix.

7. Transfer the noodles-bok choy into a serving plate. Put shredded chicken on top of the noodles. Pour peanut sauce

over the chicken and noodles. Drizzle everything with sesame oil. Serve with a sprinkle of sesame seeds and scallions.

Nutrition information

Per serving size: about 1⅔ cups

- 473 calories
- 50 g carbohydrates
- 0 g added sugars
- 2 g sugars
- 5 g fiber
- 19 g fat (3 g saturated fat)
- 26 mg cholesterol
- 23 g protein
- 280 mg sodium
- 3,261 IU vitamin A
- 204 mcg folate
- 4 mg iron
- 127 mg calcium

Creamy Mustard Chicken

4 servings

Ingredients

- 4 thin chicken breasts slices or cutlets
- ½ package whole-wheat angel hair pasta
- ½ teaspoon garlic powder
- ½ teaspoon freshly ground pepper, divided
- ½ teaspoon salt, divided
- ¼ cup all-purpose flour
- 1 large shallot, chopped finely
- 3 tablespoons extra-virgin olive oil, divided
- ½ cup water
- ½ cup dry white wine
- 2 tablespoons Dijon mustard
- ¼ cup reduced-fat sour cream
- 2 tablespoons chopped fresh sage, add a few more for garnish

Make

1. Boil water enough to cook pasta in a large pot. Follow the package directions to cook the pasta. Drain once cooked and rinse with cold water. Drain well and set aside.

2. Season chicken with ¼ teaspoon pepper and salt. Add garlic powder and mix.

3. Put flour in a shallow dish. Coat the chicken on all sides with flour. Shake to remove excess flour. Set aside on a plate. Once

all the chicken has been floured, keep 2 tablespoons of the remaining flour and discard the rest.

4. Put oil in a skillet and heat over medium high setting on a stove. Cook chicken until all sides are browned, flipping once for even cooking. Place cooked chicken on a clean plate. Lower the heat once all the chicken is cooked.

5. Pour the remaining 1 tablespoon oil into the skillet. Lower heat setting to medium. Sauté the shallot, stirring until it starts to brown. Pour wine into the skillet and stir once. Continue cooking for another minute. Mix a few tablespoons of water to the reserved dredging flour. Mix well until evenly combined. Add into the skillet. Stir and cook until the sauce thickens. Turn off the heat.

6. Stir in mustard, sage, sour cream, and ¼ teaspoon each of pepper and salt. Add chicken into the skillet. Stir to coat the chicken with the sauce.

7. Place pasta on a serving plate. Scoop half of the sauce and pour over the pasta. Spoon some of the chicken over the sauce. Pour the remaining sauce over the chicken. Serve with a garnish of sage.

Nutrition information

Per serving size: 1 chicken cutlet, 1 cup pasta & ¼ cup sauce

- 447 calories
- 42 g carbohydrates

- 6 g fiber
- 0 g added sugars
- 2 g sugars
- 16 g fat (3 g saturated fat)
- 68 mg cholesterol
- 31 g protein
- 463 mg sodium
- 154 IU vitamin A
- 41 mcg folate
- 1 mg vitamin C
- 3 mg iron
- 60 mg calcium
- 367 mg potassium

Smoky Black Bean Soup

6 servings

Ingredients

- 2 cups dried black beans
- 2 tablespoons extra-virgin olive oil
- 1 red bell pepper, chopped finely
- 2 medium onions, chopped finely, reserve ⅓ cup for garnish
- 2 large celery stalks, chopped
- 3 large garlic cloves, minced
- 1 jalapeño pepper, seeds discarded, flesh chopped finely
- 1 tablespoon ground cumin
- 2 cups brewed coffee
- 4 cups water
- 1 bay leaf
- 1 ham hock
- 1 teaspoon salt, add more as needed
- 6 tablespoons plain Greek yogurt or reduced-fat sour cream, for serving
- fresh chopped cilantro for garnish

Make

1. Rinse beans well then soak in 2 inches of water for 6 hours to overnight. Drain.

2. Pour oil into a Dutch oven or large soup pot and heat over medium high. Put onions in but reserve 1/3 cup for garnish.

Sauté together with jalapeno, garlic, celery and bell pepper. Cook vegetables for 5 to 8 minutes until starting to become fragrant. Put cumin into the pot and cook for another minute. Add coffee, water, beans, bay leaf and ham hock. Cover the pot and let the soup boil. Lower the heat to just a simmer. Remove any foam that forms on the surface of the soup. Lower heat setting to a simmer. Cook until the beans become very tender. This will take around 1 ¼ to 1 ½ hours. Once beans are done, remove bay leaf and discard. Remove ham hock also and set aside. Season with salt.

3. Pour half of the soup into a food processor. Be careful. Pulse until smooth. Pour the puree back into the pot. Return the pot to heat. Cook until the soup is heated through.

4. Slice the meat from the ham hock. Remove any fat. Slice meat into small pieces. Return the meat into the soup.

5. Ladle soup into serving bowls. Serve with a dollop of yogurt or sour cream, sprinkled with cilantro and chopped onions.

Nutrition information

Per serving size: 1⅓ cups

- 297 calories
- 43 g carbohydrates
- 15 g fiber
- 0 g added sugars
- 3 g sugars

- 8 g fat (2 g saturated fat)
- 6 mg cholesterol
- 15 g protein
- 430 mg sodium
- 811 IU vitamin A
- 257 mcg folate
- 32 mg vitamin C
- 4 mg iron
- 92 mg calcium
- 769 mg potassium

CHAPTER 6

SNACK DASH RECIPES

Berry Nut Parfait

1 serving

Ingredients

- 1 cup plain nonfat Greek yogurt
- ¼ cup frozen or fresh blueberries
- ¼ cup frozen or fresh raspberries
- 2 teaspoons honey
- ¼ cup sliced toasted almonds

Make

1. Create separate layers for each of the ingredients. Start with a layer of yogurt followed by raspberries, then a layer of the toasted almonds.

2. Add another yogurt layer.

3. Add a layer of blueberries. Add another layer of almonds then of yogurt.

4. Sprinkle remaining almonds and drizzle with honey.

5. Serve chilled.

Nutrition information

Per serving size: 1⅔ cups

- 378 calories
- 35 g carbohydrates
- 6 g fiber
- 12 g added sugars
- 25 g sugars
- 15 g fat (1 g saturated fat)
- 11 mg cholesterol
- 30 g protein
- 83 mg sodium
- 40 IU vitamin A
- 37 mcg folate
- 12 mg vitamin C
- 2 mg iron
- 336 mg calcium
- 610 mg potassium

Simple Healthy Granola Bars

Serves: 10 bars

Ingredients

- 1 cup unsalted roasted almonds, chopped loosely
- 1 packed heaping cup pitted dates
- 1/4 cup almond butter creamy or natural salted peanut butter
- 1/4 cup maple syrup, honey or agave nectar
- 1 1/2 cups rolled oats

<u>Optional additions</u>

- banana chips
- chocolate chips
- nuts
- dried fruit
- vanilla

Make

1. Place dates inside a blender or a food processor and process until it becomes like dough. Transfer the dates into a large bowl. Add almonds and oats into the bowl.

2. Place a small saucepan on a stove set on low heat. Add peanut butter and honey. Heat the mixture then pour into the bowl with the oats mixture. Stir to mix everything in the bowl. Break the dates up for even mixing. Transfer the mixture into parchment-lined 8-by-8 inches baking dish.

3. Press down on the mixture firmly until it is evenly distributed and flattened inside the baking dish. Pack the mixture really nice to have granola bars that hold well together. Chill the granola for 15 to 20 minutes until it becomes firm.

4. Lift the edges of the parchment paper to remove the granola from the pan. Transfer to a chopping board.

5. Slice into 10 bars.

Nutrition Information

Per serving size: one bar

- 217 calories
- 8 g fat (1 g saturated fat)
- 31 g carbohydrates
- 4 g fiber
- 19 g sugar
- 6 g protein

Chia Chocolate Pudding Parfaits

4 parfaits

Ingredients

Chocolate chia pudding

- 6 tablespoons chia seeds
- 2 tablespoons unsweetened cocoa powder
- 2 cups unsweetened almond milk
- 1 teaspoon ground cinnamon
- 1 teaspoon vanilla extract
- 3 tablespoons maple syrup

Mango Mousse

- 1 cup mango chunks
- 8 ounces silken tofu
- 1 tablespoon maple syrup

Mixed Berry Mousse

- 8 ounces silken tofu
- 3/4 cup (about 4 to 5 large pieces) strawberries
- 3/4 cup raspberries
- 1 1/2 tablespoons maple syrup

Toppings

- raspberries
- sliced strawberries

- pumpkin seeds
- shredded coconut

Make

1. Fill 2 medium-sized wide-mouthed jars with 1 tablespoon cocoa powder, ½ teaspoon cinnamon and 3 tablespoon chia seeds. Pour 1 cup almond milk into each of the jar. Stir the contents of the jars with a fork. Set the jars aside for 15 minutes to let the chia seeds sit for a while.

2. Stir the chia mixture again and break up any clumps of cocoa powder or chia seeds. Chill in the refrigerator for 4 hours to overnight. Check if the chia seeds have become plump. Add ½ teaspoon vanilla and 1 ½ tablespoons maple syrup. Stir.

3. Put all the ingredients for the mango mousse in a food processor. Pulse to turn it into a smooth mixture. Adjust the sweetness by adding 1 to 2 teaspoons more of maple syrup. Transfer the mousse into a large bowl. Rinse the blade and bowl of the food processor.

4. Put all the ingredients for the berry mouse. Pulse until it turns into a smooth mixture. Adjust the sweetness by adding more maple syrup as desired. Transfer the berry mousse into large bowl.

5. Divide the chia pudding mixture between 4 small jars. Divide the mango mousse between the jars. Divide the berry mousse

between the jars. Top each jar with sliced raspberries and strawberries.

6. Place shredded coconut over the fruits and sprinkle some pumpkin seeds. Serve.

Nutrition information

Per serving size: 1 glass

- 309 calories
- 41.3 g carbohydrate
- 25 g sugar
- 12.5 g fiber
- 12.3 g fat (2.3 g saturated fat)
- 0 mg cholesterol
- 14.3 g protein
- 107 mg sodium

Chili Mango Snack Bars

10 bars servings

Ingredients

- 1 cup crispy rice cereal
- 1 cup rolled oats
- 2/3 cup chopped dried mango
- 1/2 cup raw almonds
- 1/3 cup pumpkin seeds
- 3/4 teaspoon red pepper flakes
- 1/4 cup almond butter
- 2/3 cup brown rice syrup
- 1 teaspoon vanilla extract

Make

1. Prepare the oven temperature to 325F. Place one rack in the upper third position and another in the lower third position. Place parchment paper over a large cookie or baking sheet. Spread the oats in a single layer over the lined baking sheet.

2. Get a pie dish. Spread almonds in an even layer on this pie dish. Place the baking sheet with the oats in the lower rack. Place the pie dish with the almonds in the upper rack. Bake both for 10 minutes. Remove the oats and the almonds from the oven. Cool slightly.

3. Get an 8-x-8-inch pan. Line it with parchment paper. Place almonds, oats, cereals, pumpkin seeds, red pepper flakes and

mango in a mixing bowl. Heat almond butter and brown rice syrup over medium heat. Allow the mixture to start to bubble before stirring together. Lower the heat setting to low. Cook while stirring until the mixture turns into a smooth sauce. Remove the mixture from heat.

4.   Add vanilla into the sauce and stir. Pour this sauce into the bowl with the almond-oat mixture. Stir to combine into an even mixture.

5.   Transfer the mixture into the parchment paper-lined baking pan. Press down on the mixture and spread it flat and even. Press down to pack the mixture tightly.

6.   Chill or set aside at room temperature until the mixture cools and sets. Slice into 10 bars.

Nutritional information

Per serving size: 1 bar

- 219 calories
- 33.5 g carbohydrate
- 3 g fiber
- 17.6 g sugar
- 8.5 g fat (1 g saturated fat)
- 0 mg cholesterol
- 4.6 mg sodium
- 5 g protein

Strawberry Yogurt Parfait

1 serving

Ingredients

- 1 cup sliced fresh strawberries
- ½ cup plain nonfat Greek yogurt
- 1 teaspoon sugar
- ¼ cup granola

Make

1. Place sugar and strawberries in a bowl. Give a quick stir and set aside. Allow the strawberries to release its juices.

2. Layer the parfait, starting with the yogurt then the strawberries. Pour the juice in as well.

3. Top with granola and serve.

Nutrition information

Per serving size: 1½ cups

- 285 calories
- 37 g carbohydrates
- 6 g fiber
- 7 g added sugars
- 22 g sugars

- 8 g fat (1 g saturated fat)
- 6 mg cholesterol
- 17 g protein
- 50 mg sodium
- 30 IU vitamin A
- 73 mcg folate
- 98 mg vitamin C
- 2 mg iron
- 174 mg calcium
- 577 mg potassium

Mushroom Caps Stuffed with Basil Pesto

20 servings

Ingredients

- 20 cremini mushrooms, rinsed well, stems removed
- 1/4 cup melted butter
- 1 1/2 cups panko breadcrumbs
- 3 tablespoons chopped fresh parsley

Filling:

- 2 cups fresh basil leaves
- 2 tablespoons pumpkin seeds
- 1/4 cup fresh Parmesan cheese
- 1 tablespoon olive oil
- 2 teaspoons lemon juice
- 1 tablespoon fresh garlic
- 1/2 teaspoon salt

Make

1. Prepare oven temperature to 350F. Place mushroom caps on a baking sheet, upside down.

2. Mix butter, parsley and panko in a bowl. Set aside.

3. Put pumpkin seeds, lemon juice, salt, oil, cheese, garlic and basil in a food processor. Pulse until a smooth mixture is formed. Fill each mushroom cap with the filling. Sprinkle

toppings and gently pat down to keep it from falling off.

4. Bake the stuffed caps until golden brown, about 10 to 15 minutes.

5. Serve while still warm.

Nutritional information

Per serving size: 1 mushroom

- 59 calories
- 3 g fat (2 g saturated fat)
- 7 mg cholesterol
- 4 g carbohydrates
- 0 g fiber
- 0 g sugars
- 80 mg sodium
- 2 g protein

Nutty Fruit Bar

24 servings

Ingredients

- 1/2 cup quinoa flour
- 1/4 cup flax meal
- 1/2 cup oats
- 1/4 cup wheat germ
- 1/4 cup dried apricots
- 1/4 cup chopped almonds
- 1/4 cup chopped dried figs
- 1/4 cup chopped dried pineapple
- 1/4 cup buckwheat honey
- 2 tablespoons cornstarch

Make

1. Prepare the oven temperature to 300F.

2. Put all ingredients in a bowl. Stir to mix well.

3. Line a sheet pan with parchment paper. Spread the nut-fruit mixture into an even layer on the prepared sheet pan.

4. Bake for 20 minutes. Remove from oven and cool before slicing.

5. Slice into 24 bars.

Nutritional information

Per serving size: 1 bar

- 61 calories
- 11 g carbohydrates
- 1 g fiber
- 7 g added sugar
- 1 g fat (trace amounts of saturated fat)
- 0 mg cholesterol
- 5 mg sodium
- 2 g protein

CHAPTER 7

SAMPLE 7-DAY DASH DIET MEAL PLAN

Here is a simple example of how a 7-day meal plan following the DASH guidelines will look like:

Sample 7-day Diet Plan for Phase 1

<u>Day 1</u>

Breakfast

- 1 to 2 slices Canadian bacon
- Hard-boiled egg
- 6 ounces low-sodium tomato juice

Midmorning Snack

- Baby carrots
- 1 stick light cheese

Lunch

- Meatless quinoa balls
- Cherry tomatoes dressed with oil-vinegar or Italian dressing
- Strawberry sugar-free Jell-O cup

Midafternoon Snack

- 18 cashews (about 1/4 cup)
- 4 ounces light lemon fat-free, yogurt

Dinner

- Mediterranean-style chicken kabobs
- 1 cup mixed carrots, broccoli, and cauliflower with Romaine and Italian dressing
- Raspberry sugar-free Jell-O cup

Day 2

Breakfast

- Egg Beaters Southwestern Style omelet
- 4-6 ounces low-sodium tomato juice

Midmorning Snack

- 1 wedge light cheese
- 6 grape tomatoes

Lunch

- 2-3 Turkey-and-Cheese Swiss roll-ups
- 1/2-1 cup coleslaw
- Orange sugar-free Jell-O cup

Dinner

- Sliced roasted turkey
- Salad with carrots and onions drizzled with Italian dressing
- Lime sugar-free Jell-O cup

<u>Day 3</u>

Breakfast

- Scrambled eggs
- 4-6 ounces diet cranberry juice
- 1-2 slices Canadian bacon

Midmorning Snack

- 4 ounces nonfat light raspberry yogurt
- 23 almonds (about 1/4 cup)

Lunch

- Cold fried chicken breast
- Baby carrots and coleslaw
- Lemon sugar-free Jell-O cup

Midafternoon Snack

- 1-2 wedges light cheese
- 6 grape tomatoes

Dinner

- Turkey burger
- 1 cup broccoli with balsamic dressing
- 1-2 strawberry sugar-free Jell-O cups

Day 4

Breakfast

- Vegetable omelet
- 1 cup milk

Midmorning Snack

- 1/3 cup almonds, unsalted
- 1/2 cup fat-free fruit yogurt

Lunch

- 3/4 cup chicken salad
- 1 cup fresh salad with 1/2 cup fresh cucumber slices, 1/2 cup tomato wedges and 1 tablespoon sunflower seeds
- 1 teaspoon low calorie Italian dressing
- 1 cup vegetable juice

Midafternoon Snack

- 1 cup fat-free fruit yogurt

Dinner

- 3 oz. beef, eye of the round, pan seared
- 2 tablespoons fat-free beef gravy
- 1 cup sautéed green beans
- 1 cup low-fat milk

Day 5

Breakfast

- Cheesy scrambled eggs
- 1 cup fat-free milk

Midmorning Snack

- 1 cup low-fat chocolate milk

Lunch

- Sugar snap peas stir fry with diced tofu and tamari sauce
- 1 cup low-fat frozen yogurt

Midafternoon Snack

- 1 cup crispy kale chips

Dinner

- Sesame-ginger grilled salmon
- 1 cup artichoke heart salad
- 1 cup fat-free milk

Day 6

Breakfast

- 1 cup green smoothie with spinach, kale, honey and a squeeze of lemon juice

Midmorning Snack

- 1 cup toasted almonds
- 1 cup frozen yogurt

Lunch

- 1 ½ cups mushroom and spinach salad with 1 tablespoon vinaigrette dressing
- 1 cup green juice

Midafternoon Snack

- 1 stick light cheese

Dinner

- Escarole with mint and baked potatoes
- ½ cup low-fat frozen yogurt

Day 7

Breakfast

- 1 cup decaf iced coffee latte with fat-free milk
- 2 slices bacon
- 1 hard-boiled egg

Midmorning Snack

- Baked potato skins

Lunch

- Lentil salad with arugula, feta and tomatoes
- 1 cup green spinach-kale smoothie with low-fat yogurt

Midafternoon Snack

- Toasted sunflower seeds
- Fat-free yogurt
- 1 slice light cheese

Dinner

- Tuscan chicken
- Spicy orange and cucumber salad
- 1 cup cold green smoothie

Sample 7-day Diet Plan for Phase 2

Day 1

Breakfast

- 3/4 cup Wheaties
- 4-6 ounces raspberries or strawberries
- 8 ounces skim milk

Midmorning Snack

- 1-2 wedges light cheese
- Grape tomatoes

Lunch

- 2-3 turkey and Swiss roll-ups
- Small plum
- Baby carrots

Midafternoon Snack

- 10 cashews
- 6 ounces light blueberry yogurt

Before-Dinner Snack

- 10 peanuts in the shell

Dinner

- Pan-seared tilapia
- Fresh asparagus
- Mango-Melon Salsa
- Strawberry Jell-O-O cup, sugar-free

<u>Day 2</u>

Breakfast

- Hot chocolate
- 1-2 hard-boiled eggs

- 6-8 ounces light cranberry juice
- 4-6 ounces strawberries

Midmorning Snack (Optional)

- 10 ounces almonds
- 6 ounces key lime light nonfat yogurt

Lunch

- Turkey and Swiss sandwich
- Pepper strips with coleslaw
- Raspberry JellO cup

Midafternoon Snack

- 1-2 wedges light cheese
- 1 clementine orange

Before-Dinner Snack

- Pepper strips with ¼ to 1/2 cup hummus

Dinner

- Quinoa and vegetable stir fry
- Salad with Italian, or vinaigrette dressing
- Fudge bar

Day 3

Breakfast

- 1/2 cup cooked oatmeal with cinnamon, honey and 1 tablespoon chopped almonds
- 1/2 medium or large banana
- Latte made with 2 ounces espresso and 8 ounces skim milk
- 4-6 ounces low-sodium tomato juice

Midmorning Snack

- Baby carrots
- 1 stick light cheese

Lunch

- Three-Bean kale sauté with brown rice and sliced bell peppers
- Orange Jell-O-O cup

Midafternoon Snack

- 10 cashews
- 4-6 ounces strawberries

Before-Dinner Snack

- 10 peanuts in the shell

Dinner

- Cabbage and white bean soup
- Green beans and sliced tomatoes with Italian dressing
- 4-6 ounces raspberries

Day 4

Breakfast

- 1 slice whole-wheat toast
- 1-3 scrambled eggs
- 1 tablespoon jelly or jam
- Latte or 8 ounces skim milk
- 4-6 ounces orange juice

Midmorning Snack (Optional)

- 10 almonds
- 4-6 ounces blueberries

Lunch

- 2-3 roast beef with Muenster cheese roll-ups
- Italian coleslaw
- Small peach

Midafternoon Snack

- 6 ounces light strawberry yogurt

Before-Dinner Snack

- Baby carrots with 2 tablespoons peanut butter

Dinner

- Salmon-stuffed Avocado
- Lettuce, red cabbage grape tomatoes, and blue cheese crumbles with vinaigrette dressing
- Fudge bar or low-fat, low-sugar, low-calorie, ice cream bar

<u>Day 5</u>

Breakfast

- 1/2 cup oatmeal with 1 teaspoon cinnamon
- 1 cup low-fat milk

Midmorning Snack

- 1 mini whole wheat bagel
- 1 medium banana
- 1 tablespoon peanut butter

Lunch

- Chicken sandwich with : 2 slices whole wheat bread, 3 oz. skinless chicken breast, 1 slice natural low sodium Swiss cheese, 1 slice natural reduced fat cheddar cheese, 2 slices tomato, 1 large leaf romaine lettuce, 1 tablespoon low-fat mayonnaise

- 1 cup cantaloupe chunks
- 1 cup apple juice

Midafternoon Snack

- 1/3 cup almonds
- 1/4 cup raisins

Dinner

- 3 oz. cod
- 1/2 cup brown rice
- 1 cup spinach with 1 tablespoon slivered almonds
- 1 small cornbread muffin

Day 6

Breakfast

- 1 slice whole wheat bread
- 1 tsp soft unsalted margarine
- 1 medium peach
- 1 cup fat-free fruit yogurt
- 1/2 cup grape juice

Midmorning Snack

- 1/3 cup unsalted almonds
- 1/4 cup apricots
- 1 cup apple juice
- 1 cup low-fat milk

Lunch

- 1/2 cup tuna salad with 1 large leaf romaine lettuce over 1 slice whole wheat bread
- cucumber salad made with 1 cup fresh cucumber slices and 1/2 cup tomato wedges with 1 tablespoon vinaigrette dressing
- 1/2 cup canned pineapple juice

Midafternoon Snack

- 1 cup fat-free fruit yogurt
- 2 large graham cracker rectangles
- 1 tablespoon unsalted sunflower seeds
- 1 tablespoon peanut butter

Dinner

- 1 cup green peas
- Chicken and Spanish rice
- 1 cup cantaloupe chunks
- 1 cup low-fat milk

Day 7

Breakfast

- 1 cup whole grain oat rings cereal
- 1 medium raisin bagel
- 1 tablespoon unsalted peanut butter
- 1 cup orange juice

Midmorning Snack

- 1 cup fat-free fruit yogurt
- 2 tablespoons unsalted sunflower seeds

Lunch

- 3 oz. turkey meatloaf
- 1 small baked potato
- 1 tablespoon natural cheddar cheese
- 1 tablespoon sour cream, fat-free 21 1
- 1 small whole wheat roll
- 1 medium peach

Midafternoon Snack

- 2 tablespoons unsalted peanuts
- 1/4 cup dried apricots
- 1 cup low-fat milk

Dinner

- zucchini lasagna
- fresh spinach salad with 1 cup tomato wedges and 2 tablespoons croutons, seasoned with 1 tablespoon vinaigrette dressing
- 1 small whole wheat roll
- 1 cup grape juice

CONCLUSION

Thank you again for purchasing this book!

I hope this book was able to help you understand what DASH diet can do for your weight loss goals.

The next step is to make that change. Throw away everything that keeps you unhealthy like everything with high sodium content. Start shopping DASH and eat DASH from now on. Use the recipes in this book to start adapting a lifestyle that will make you healthier and look good.

Finally, if you enjoyed this book, please take the time to share your thoughts and post a review on Amazon. It'd be greatly appreciated!

In case you have forgotten, visit our website at http://www. weightlossbonusguide.com/ to grab your free bonus as it will help you further improve your health and your life. You will will be part of our VIP Inner Circle of readers and you will be able to receive all of my new books at a discounted price

Thank you and good luck!

Anne